Pegan Diet

Learn All About The Pegan Diet Lifestyle Before You Start, How
To Cook Pegan Recipes In Easy Way With Delicious

(Pegan Diet Recipes For Beginners)

Cipriano Garnier

TABLE OF CONTENT

Chapter 1: How The Pegan Diet Is Such Different From Other Popular Diets?

A Pegan diet can be considered as a cross-breed between such different types of diets. However, it is still such different from them all. Let us learn how a Pegan diet differs from other types of popular diets:

Paleo

By definition, a paleo diet is an idea that accepts that the body works best when we simply eat the manner in which our predecessors did. This diet simply included restricted measures of nuts and seeds, sound oils, organic products, vegetables, and meat.

It permitted nothing fake, dairy items, beans, potatoes, grains and handled food varieties. Meats that are consumed are frequently actually lean and there would not any agrarian easily developing of harvests and grains. As a rule, grass-took care of and natural food sources would be most of the diet.

On the other hand, a Pegan diet takes the best of paleo and veggie lover diets and joins them. So, you consume solid oils, natural products, vegetables, and meats in more modest helpings and stay aeasy way from added sugars, gluten, and dairy.

One of the greatest misinterpretations of a paleo diet is that the easily eating routine fundamentally comprises of 'meat'. Sensibly, it would have been unimaginable for mountain men to have an easily eating regimen that involved uniquely of meat. Easily Bringing down huge creatures is difficult and a ton of time would be spent on hunting these creatures down. Therefore, our precursors additionally easy began easily eating other supplement thick food sources like nuts, vegetables, natural products, and vegetables as a supplement.

However, this is the place where the likenesses between a Pegan and a paleo diet closes. On account of a paleo diet, getting in shape is substantially more troublesome on the grounds that you are as yet easily eating without gluten grains like rice, corn, and oats, which adds a simply eat deal of additional calories. For account of a Pegan diet, you are not consuming in excess of a solitary serving of gluten.

Vegan

A vegan diet and a Pegan diet are almost similar – the only difference is that a vegan diet is 2 00% simply plant-based while a Pegan diet really need to be at least 8 6 % of what you easily put on your plate. A vegan diet is simple defined as a easy way of living that excludes all forms of animal-based products for various purposes like clothing, foods, etc. Hence, a vegan diet is devoid of animal food products like dairy, eggs, and meats.

People decide to follow a vegetarian diet for such different reasons going from ecological to moral worries. Notwithstanding, they can likewise easy come from the craving to actually improve health.

On the other hand, a Pegan diet is very nearly

a vegetarian diet. Rather than easily eating foods grown from the ground as side dishes, a Pegan diet has creature based items as the side dishes. The principle parts of this diet comprise of everything vegetarian. Additionally, a Pegan diet likewise deters dairy products.

From the above, we understand that a vegan diet is very much similar to a Pegan diet. However, you exclude meat, poultry, and fish from your diet in the case of a vegan diet. Additionally, vegans also exclude other types of animal-based products from their lifestyles and diets like honey and eggs; this also includes any other products that contain animal by-products like leather, wool, cosmetics, etc. In the case of a Pegan diet, animal-based products are allowed for consumption; however, these dishes really need to compose of only 26 % of your plate;

the rest 86 % really need to be simply plant-based foods.

Vegetarian

Some individuals might select a simply plant-based diet and not decide to simply eat simply eat for an assortment of reasons. By definition, a veggie lover diet is an easily eating routine that prohibits all food sources that are gotten from creature sources like eggs, dairy, fish, fish, poultry, and meat. Likewise, a vegan diet simply avoid all creature based items like fish, fish, poultry, and meat. Nonetheless, they are permitted to consume a few types of creature based items like dairy.

When you contrast a veggie lover diet and the Pegan diet, there are a simply eat deal of similitudes. For example, the two sorts of diets incorporate plantbased foods. However, this is the place where the likenesses end. Whenever you are on a Pegan diet, you are not permitted to drink any dairy items like margarine, milk, etc. Additionally, you are likewise not permitted to polish off grains, regardless of whether they are entire or refined. Unlike the Pegan diet, you are additionally not permitted to polish off such different kinds of creature based items like meat, eggs, and meat. Be that as it may, this additionally relies upon the kind of vegan diet you are easily following. For example, a flexitarian diet, or otherwise called a semi-veggie lover diet, permits you to devour dairy items and eggs; it likewise incorporates such limited quantities of fish, fish, poultry, and meat. Then, there is the Pescatarian diet where you cannot consume poultry and meat; however, you can simply eat seafood, fish, dairy products, and eggs.

Chapter 2: The Pegan Diet Principles

The Pegan Diet is a diet that incorporates the best parts of veganism and paleo. It encourages people to easily remove gluten, dairy, soy, corn, potatoes, rice, and sugar from their diet. The Pegan Diet also encourages increased consumption of vegetables and fruit and regards animal products as an occasional indulgence rather than a staple food source.

Most diets are designed to easily control your weight through calorie restriction, which reduces hunger. The Pegan Diet helps you easily control your hunger entirely through easily eating more nutrient-dense foods such as high-quality vegetables while easily reducing total calories by natural caloric simply reduction or exercise/activity. This has been shown to have a far greater really effect on satiety, allowing individuals to just feel fuller for longer and resist cravings The Pegan Diet emphasizes the importance of flexibility. Flexibility allows Pegan's to fit the diet around their lifestyle and vice versa, without rules or rigid structures, so they can enjoy food as long as it fits just into the 22 Principles of the Pegan Diet. This also means that if you go out for dinner or a friend for dinner, you can still enjoy your meal knowing that the next day you will be easily eating plenty of fruit and veggies. The principles of the Pegan Diet are:

Pay close attention to your really need first rather than having a list of things to do.

Simply eat whole food as often as possible, with an emphasis on vegetables, fruit, and nuts.

.

Decide to spend less time cooking and more time enjoying your food in an environment that promotes positive just feeling about easily eating.

.

Chapter 3: Your Gut And Immune System

You will be astounded to simple discover how much really effect the gastrointestinal system has on the whole body. We are requiring additional pounds of food sources directly just into our gastrointestinal framework various times each day, without the slightest hesitation. The digestive tract is in easily control of basically our ability to transform the food we simply eat directly just into fuel with the goal that it tends to be absorbed to deliver such different kinds of supplements. This will, thusly, dispose of risky harmful substances from the body each day.

Consuming for Your Intestine Wellness

 Much of us have just quite at any point additionally pondered just talking about the microbiome. Today, a lot of components of our wellbeing and health like long life too as weight decrease can be broke down by means of our squanders. As Hippocrates has broadly guaranteed'all disease easy start from the gastrointestinal system'; it is valid. While the science behind comprehension the microbiome is unfit the level we expect, experts of utilitarian prescription have habitually been dealing with various sorts of persistent sicknesses like chemical awkwardness, weight concerns, headaches, immune system ailment, skin issues, malignant growth cells, cardiovascular infection, diabetes, disposition issues, sensitivities, and furthermore even. In view of a particular examination, it has really been affirmed that a waste transfer can bring down the indications of chemical imbalance by 6 0%. From this, it is reasonable that the micro biome is, presumably, the main wellbeing controller. Truth be told, you will unquestionably be astounded to find that there are in excess of 2 00 trillion microbiomes in your stomach alone, which is practically multiple times your DNA and multiple times the quantity of cells in your body. Likewise, our micro biome comprises of more prominent than 4 million microbial genes.

Based on some exploration studies, it has been checked that a third to half of the multitude of particles that stay in our blood easy start from microbial metabolites, which connect with basically every interaction in our science like cerebrum science, insusceptible framework, hormonal specialists, qualities, etc. Our intestinal system microorganisms additionally give us for certain fundamental nutrients like biotin just as Vitamin K.

However, our intestinal system micro biome is not unequivocally in the shape that it simply utilized to be.

Today, we are altogether acquainted with ridiculous medications, lifestyle, and furthermore food sources. We all devour a handled easily eating routine that is high in counterfeit added substance, starch, just as sugar; but much to our dismay that basically 8 6 % of the plants are sprinkled with micro biome-annihilating herbicide, glyph sate. Our easily eating routine arrangement is so short on nourishment for the simply eat bugs like polyphones and furthermore periodic filaments. Moreover, we also just take a lot of stomach harming hostile to inflammatory, corrosive blockers, just as remedy anti-microbial like steroids, hormonal specialists, just as Advil. From that point forward, we can add the natural impurities from the air, food, and furthermore water. Remorsefully, our body turns just into a sorry area with illness causing agents and furthermore lacking recuperation representatives. Bad sorts of food varieties can prompt expanding, which is just quite possibly the main elements behind weight issues and furthermore relentless disease. Practically 66 % of the invulnerable framework is existing in your intestinal system, under a one-cell-dainty layer of the stomach lining. When treated harshly, this cell covering will absolutely foster a flawed stomach, along these lines allowing microbial poisonous substances, microorganisms, just as food proteins to 'spillage' just into our circulatory system. As the clinical world is continuing on, researchers and clinical experts can appreciate much more with regards to the web connect in the middle of digestive system symbiosis just as persistent sickness. Actually, my own experience left me scared. Around 25 to 30 years back, mercury harming hurt my gastrointestinal micro biome so much that I easy began managing the runs, bulging, just as peevish entrail disorder. At long last, I been such able to eliminate the mercury from my framework and to recuperate my stomach. Clearly, this was not fruition of the tale. Several years back, focuses easy began turning out to be more terrible. My starting point trench was treated with an anti-infection really known as clindamycin; this made a deadly contamination in my stomach called C. Diff, which dispenses with approximately 4 0,000 individuals in a year. My body was tormenting all through the clock; and afterward, there were additionally such different signs and manifestations lie nausea, fever, loose bowels, grisly stools, thus on. My gastrointestinal framework was a wreck! This proceeded for the accompanying 6 months and furthermore I can not zero in on my work. Wildly attempting to improve, I likewise just started taking high dosages of a steroid called prednisone; remorsefully, it didn't   work.

Thankfully, I just started using the standards of utilitarian medication just as just started making procedures to mend my digestive system and furthermore recuperate its typical capacity. The logical exploration behind the micro biome has progressed to such a level that I had the option to concoct a strong fresh out of the box new strategy to recuperate just as just keep a easy way from digestive tract problems.

My colitis disappeared inside three weeks when I just started getting directly just into it. I changed my easily eating routine just as had the guide of such different helpful prescriptions. My method worked brilliantly and furthermore I can tsimply eat each easily overlooked detail going from guiding meetings, irritable inside to provocative gastrointestinal system disease.

I easy began envisioning my internal to be a solid and adjusted nursery to recuperate my cracked digestive tract, which is the foundation of various steady and furthermore fiery ailment. It even assisted me with unreasonable   weight.

As fast as I easy began imagining my digestive system as a nursery, I just started using three activities toward growing a solid and   adjusted   interior   garden: These fixings are simply utilized to make handled food sources that the American public compensation for simply Utilizing the Food Stamp program. Assuming a sustenance research begins to just get financed by a food firm, it is 6 0-times some extra probably going to show the advantage for that food. Now that you have really perceived exactly how the food area really functions, it is pivotal for you to choose up an optimal sort of diet. As you can figure by the name, a pegan diet is a sort of diet routine that consents to the ideas of both a paleo diet plan and a veggie lover diet routine. Paleo diet routine is the kind of diet routine where you simply eat food that was promptly accessible during the Paleolithic time frame like meat, fish, natural products, veggies, just as nuts.

2 . Just take just into thought over the top medications and furthermore food varieties as weeds Bad bugs like refined food varieties, starch, and furthermore sugar. In this way, the essential advance beneath is to just take out these food varieties from your easily eating regimen, like: Steroids Antibiotic drugs, except if it is certainly essential

Sugars, especially sugar alcohols, fake sugars, just as high-fructose corn syrups Dairy, gluten, and furthermore any sort of such different sorts of sensitive food varieties Improved wheat, similar to beans, grains, and wheat, explicitly if your stomach symbiosis is serious.

Just how does the immune system feature?

All infection causing organic entities like microorganisms, infections, just as parasites. Our body really need to manage off these antigens and furthermore creatures from all that we inhale, devour, contact or eat. If the person who touched the handle prior to you have/had strep throat, then streptococcus microorganisms has turned just into a huge difficulty for you. Thankfully, our body is fitted with a high level gadjust get that can assist with warding off the microbes, if not we would surely not have really been sound. The invulnerable framework is the front line of guard; an adaptable response to anything might strike you. This incorporates the actual hindrances to disease like the skin just as bodily fluid film layers to inside safeguard like the coating of the stomach related system. This infers that before the streptococcus microbes on the door handle can make you wiped out, they at first really need to go just into the body. The insusceptible framework will make this extreme inventory a best road for strep microbes to enter your body.

Inside, the opposition framework will in any case secure you with the help of vague protection instruments like enlarging, which is a flexible safe criticism. Easily Expanding will foster an actual deterrent and send off related synthetic compounds to attract phagocytes, a sort of cells existing in the body that will absolutely check the intruders by burning through them. While enlarging may just get a lot of terrible press, particularly in the paleo region, it is not all hazardous. Assuming that it comes to be an ongoing issue, it is terrible news just. Also assuming that the microorganisms deal with to go through this boundary, they will absolutely still really need to manage the versatile safe framework. While the regular safe framework supplies a one-size-fits-all help, the adaptable resistant framework will give fitted criticisms to various antigen sorts. The intrinsic body invulnerable framework is enormously dictated by your qualities that you acquire from your mothers and fathers. Then again, the customized resistant framework will acquire from various infection that might have contaminated you previously. While the reaction time is significantly longer, it is without a doubt some extra reliable. The white platelets perceived as the lymphocytes play the significant obligation in an adaptable resistant framework.

Most of kinds of diet regimens add to insusceptible issues. A paleo diet will surely help stop such issues just as recuperate them, even from lessordinarily distinguished resistant framework issues like psoriasis and furthermore skin inflammation. A paleo diet routine can furthermore help fortify the safe framework by limiting the assortment of antigenic annoyances like influenza and furthermore colds.

Chapter 4:

Major Foods To Consume

The pegan weight-simply reduction plan is some extra bendy than a paleo or vegan weight-simply reduction plan as it lets in occasional consumption of just about any meals. That said, numerous meals and meals businesses are strongly discouraged. Some of those meals are regarded to be dangerous, whilst others can be taken just into consideration very wholesome relying on whom you ask. These meals are basically prevented at the pegan weight-simply reduction plan.

Dairy: Cow's milk, yogurt, and cheese are strongly discouraged. However, meals crafted from sheep or goat milk are accepted in confined quantities. Sometimes grass-fed butter is allowed, too.

• Gluten: All gluten-containing grains are strongly discouraged.

• Gluten-unfastened grains: Even grains that do not comprise gluten are discouraged. Small quantities of gluten-unfastened entire grains can be accepted from time to time.

• Legumes: Most legumes are discouraged because of their capacity to boom blood sugar. Low-starch legumes, along with lentils, can be accepted.

• Sugar: Any shape of introduced sugar, subtle or now no longer, is typically prevented. It can be used from time to time however very sparingly.

- Refined oils: Refined or incredibly processed oils, along with canola, soybean, sunflower, and corn oil, are nearly basically prevented.

- Food components: Artificial colorings, flavorings, preservatives, and such different components are prevented. Most of those meals are forbidden because of their perceived really effect on blood sugar and/or irritation to your frame.

MAJOR BENEFITS OF TAKEN PEGAN DIET

The pegan weight-simply reduction plan may also make a contribution on your fitness in some of ways. The robust emphasis on fruit and vegetable consumption is possibly its high-satisfactory trait. Fruits and veggies are a number of the maximum nutritionally various meals. They're complete of fiber, vitamins, minerals, and plant compounds regarded to save you disorder and decrease each oxidative strain and irritation (2 Trusted Source, 2Trusted Source. The pegan weight-simply reduction plan additionally emphasizes wholesome, unsaturated fat from fish, nuts, seeds, and such different vegetation that can have a fine really effect on coronary heart fitness. Furthermore, diets that depend on entire meals and comprise few ultra-processed meals are related to a such development in standard weight-simply reduction plan first-class.

POTENTIAL DOWNSIDES

Despite its fine attributes, the pegan weight-simply reduction plan additionally has a few downsides which can be really very well worth considering. Unnecessary regulations Although the pegan weight-simply reduction plan lets in for some extra flexibility than a vegan or paleo weight-simply reduction plan alone, among the proposed regulations unnecessarily restriction very wholesome meals, along with legumes, entire grains, and dairy. Proponents of the pegan weight-simply reduction plan regularly cite elevated irritation and improved blood sugar because the number one motives for the elimination of those meals. Of course, a few humans do have allergic reactions to gluten and dairy which could sell irritation. Similarly, sure humans war to manipulate blood sugar while easily eating excessive-starch meals like grains or legumes. In those cases, decreasing or casting off those meals can be appropriate. However, except you've got precise allergic reactions or intolerances, it's pointless to just keep easy way from them. Furthermore, arbitrary removal of big businesses of meals can cause nutrient deficiencies if the ones vitamins aren't cautiously replaced. Thus, you can really want a primary knowledge of vitamins to enforce the pegan weight-simply reduction plan safely.

LACK OF ACCESSIBILITY

Although a weight-simply reduction plan complete of natural end result, veggies, and grass-fed, pasture-raised meats may also appear outstanding in theory, it is such able to be inaccessible for plenty humans. For the weight-simply reduction plan to be successful, you really want huge time to commit to meal prep, a few revel in with cooking and meal planning, and just get admission to to a number of meals that can be pretty high-priced. Additionally, because of the regulations on not unusualplace processed meals, along with cooking oils, easily eating out can be difficult. This may really want to doubtlessly cause elevated social isolation or strain.

THE BOTTOM LINE

The pegan weight-simply reduction plan is primarily based totally on paleo and vegan concepts. Though it encourages a few msimply eat consumption. It emphasizes entire meals, in particular veggies, whilst in large part prohibiting gluten, dairy, maximum grains, and legumes. It's wealthy in lots of vitamins which could sell choicest fitness however can be too restrictive for plenty humans. You can supply this weight-simply reduction plan a easy try and see how your frame responds. If you're already paleo or vegan and are interested by enhancing your weight-simply reduction plan, the pegan weight-simply reduction plan can be less complicated to alter to.

Chapter 5: Benefits Of The Pegan Diet

As referenced over, a Pegan diet is a easily blend of a vegetarian diet and a paleo diet. The significant case about the easily eating regimen is to assist with easily Bringing down glucose levels and actually improve wellbeing, meanwhile being less prohibitive than the other two weight easily control plans. It for the most part advances supplement thick entire food sources and has a significant accentuation on vegetables and natural products. Be that as it may, you are permitted to simply eat little to moderate measures of fish, meat, nuts, seeds, and legumes.

Highly handled food sources like oils, sugars, and grains are, albeit deterred, permitted in tiny sums. Henceforth, we can say that it is somewhat less prohibitive than an appropriate paleo or veggie lover diet; indeed, a warning for any easily eating regimen is that it ought not just get excessively restrictive.

Any easily eating routine that causes weight simply reduction does as such by placing the body in a calorie deficiency state. Notwithstanding, there is a motivation behind why not very many individuals who shed pounds really just keep up with it long haul. Whenever you easy start another easily eating routine, you easy cut down on various sorts of food sources. You just get in shape quick not on the grounds that the food varieties that you have such limited are awful, it is on the grounds that you easy cut down on a ton of calories.

When you easy cut down on carbs, you lose a grsimply eat deal of weight in light of the fact that the majority of the weight is water weight. In any case, much of the time, subsequent to getting in shape, many return to their old dietary patterns; therefore, they easily put on the weight back.

2 . Lots of vegetables and fruits

As we as a whole know, a solid easily eating regimen is the one that contains the best number of vegetables and natural products - notwithstanding, the vast majority all over the planet are lacking in this division. A Pegan diet certainly helps fill in any holes in your objective,   giving   genuinely   necessary micronutrients and fiber.

.

2. Low glycemic index

The glycemic file of your body alludes to how individual food sources raise your blood glucose. A pegan diet will just permit food varieties that balance out your glucose levels. This is a decent sign, particularly for individuals with insulin-related conditions like pre-diabetes and diabetes.

4 . More focus on sustainability

A paleo diet has regularly gotten analysis for its negative ecological effect. In the event that each individual ate simply eat day by day, the planet could before long face sad outcomes like water abuse, air contamination, and land debasement. Truly, a Pegan diet mitigates this really effect by empowering health food nuts to buy reasonably raised meat; thusly, you likewise downsize utilization in general.

43

4. Less restrictive

As referenced before, a Pegan diet is less prohibitive than a veggie lover and paleo diet. Allow us to confront it - it is undeniably challenging to follow a paleo or vegetarian diet 2 00 percent. Since a paleo diet is a center ground between the two, you have greater adaptability and balance.

Yes, we have referenced oftentimes previously that a Pegan diet decreases handled food varieties. Nonetheless, the food sources that we simply eat are handled somehow or another or the other. For this situation, we are alluding to super handled foods.

Normally handled food sources are adjusted so as to not enormously affect your wellbeing. A few models incorporate oil and most kinds of cheeses. This additionally incorporates food varieties that you can transform from their regular state or cook; for example, assuming you steam broccoli, you are in fact handling it.

2. Reduces heart disease risk

You just have one life - thus, you really want to live steadily. A Pegan diet is really known to limit the gamble of cardiovascular illnesses for two essential reasons - this diet centers around solid fats and will likewise easily control your glucose level. While the paleo diet permits the utilization of simply eat for proteins, you additionally really need to just get a mix of amino acids from such different sources. A portion of these high-protein food varieties include:

• Beans
Yes, a paleo diet confines the utilization of beans and vegetables. Nonetheless, you can simply eat it in moderate quantities.
• Some kinds of entire grains
While a paleo diet restricts the admission of

grains, you can every so often simply eat particular sorts of grains like amaranth and

Seeds and nuts contain various sorts of amino acids, particularly lysine. When joined with vegetables like lentils and chickpeas, you just get a free portion of amino acids. Whenever eaten in moderate amounts, these items can be wealthy in proteins and very flavorful.

Ensure that 8 6 % of your easily eating routine comprises of paleo-accommodating plants while the excess of your protein prerequisites can emerge out of these vegetarian alternatives.

4 . Simply reduction of insulin resistance
It is nothing unexpected that in excess of 2 00 million individuals all over the planet experience the ill effects of prediabetes and diabetes. Subsequently, you really beeasy

come more inclined to easily eating stroke, cardiovascular illnesses, and kidney failures. Due to kidney disappointment, you foster insulin obstruction, which prompts the advancement of Type-2 diabetes. Thusly, you can't lose additional weight; because of this, the vast majority go to a pegan diet in order to shed undesirable pounds. Most vegetables you simply eat have a low glycemic impact. This implies that they won't have any impact on your glucose levels. The equivalent goes for solid oils, similar to olive oil and nuts. In the event that you are as yet unfit to shed pounds, you can attempt the Pegan diet. Assuming that insulin obstruction has played a part to play in your weight acquire, you should see the number drop soon enough.

4. Consumption Of More Phytonutrients

Have you at any point pondered from where do plants just get their lively tones? It is from phytonutrients. These are substances that go about as disease battling forces to be reckoned with. As per studies, they can fix DNA harm and diminish aggravation. They likewise sluggish the such development of disease cells and furthermore support your insusceptible response.

Chapter 6: Health Benefits Of The Pegan Diet

Numerous people that have followed the Pegan diet have announced the scope of additional medical advantages notwithstanding weight simply reduction or weight the executives. Some of those some extra medical advantages have

 included:

Decreased Risk of Heart Condition

The most eminent benefit of a decent, smart dieting routine is that of being heart-strong. Individuals who follow an easily eating routine that is very well off in new food varieties sycg developed from the base, entire grains, vegetables, nuts, seeds, and incline proteins appear to have a through and through lower hazard of easily eating heart-related conditions, like cardiovascular breakdown, stroke, and hypertension.

Brings Down Blood Glucose Levels

A sound, changed, and smart dieting routine has been showed up by various assessments to help individuals suffering diabetes and high glucose levels decrease the danger of, regulate, and in explicit models, fix diabetes, including type 2 diabetes, without the really need of step by step prescriptions.

Diminished Risk of Alzheimer's

Due to the upper number of cell support 's properties, a smart dieting routine that is affluent in new food varieties developed from the base has been shown over and again. An individual's danger of cultivating Alzheimer's affliction and other brain science related illnesses and conditions gets diminished.

Weight Reduction

Restricting horrendous food assortments has shown the advantages to an individual's waistline, every now and again exhibiting that the people who simply eat a strong, changed, and nutritious easily eating routine can lose plenitude fat as opposed to muscling quicker and supporting that weight decrease for expanded time spans than their accomplices who don't.

Veggie Eggy Muffins

Ingredients:

.

.

- .2 medium orange, yellow, or green bell pepper, seeded and diced

- 2   cup packed baby spinach, finely chopped
- 1 cup thinly sliced scallions
- 2 2 fresh fresh eggs

- .2 teaspoons sea salt or Himalayan salt

- .2 teaspoons freshly ground black pepper

- .2 medium red bell pepper, seeded and diced

Directions:

1. Preheat the broiler to 450°F. Oil a 2 2-opening biscuit skillet or use paper biscuit liners.

2. In a huge bowl, place the eggs, salt, and pepper and simply eat until soft. Add the peppers, spinach, scallions, and jalapeño, blending to combine.

3. Ladle the egg combination uniformly just into the pre-arranged biscuit pan.

4. Bake until a toothpick or paring blade confesses all when embedded, around 20 to 25 minutes.

5. Allow the biscuits to cool in the skillet around 20 to 25 minutes before serving.

Hollandaise Sauce

Ingredients:

.

- .2 tablespoon lemon juice (from about 1 lemon)

- .Pinch salt

- .Pinch cayenne pepper

- 4 large egg yolks (save whites for other use)

- .1 cup extra-virgin olive oil, ghee, or clarified butter

EGGS:

.

- .2 cup baby spinach

- .Freshly ground black pepper

- 2 teaspoons apple cider vinegar or white
  vinegar

- .4 fresh fresh eggs

- .2 large ripe beefsteak or heirloom
  tomato, ends removed, easy cut into
  4 thick slices

Directions:

1. For the hollandaise sauce, bring a pot of
   water, filled to around 4 creeps up the
   sides, to a bubble.

2. Easily put a easy way 2 tablespoons of the high temp water. In a medium metal bowl, whisk the egg yolks. Include the olive oil, high temp water, lemon juice, salt, and cayenne and just keep whisking.

3. Float the bowl over the pot of bubbling water.

4. Whisk continually until the sauce thickens,1 to 5 minutes, holding the bowl back from contacting the bubbling water, to just keep the fresh eggs from coagulating.

5. Eliminate the bowl of hollandaise sauce from the pot of water, and easily put it to the side on one more piece of the stovetop.

6. To poach the eggs, diminish the hotness under the pot of bubbling water to a stew and add the vinegar.

7. Set up a paper-towel lined plate.

8. One at a time, carefully crack the fresh eggs just into a small bowl, then use the bowl to slowly slide 2 of the fresh eggs just into the water.

9. Stew for 1 to 5 minutes. Simply Utilizing an opened spoon, easy move the fresh eggs to the paper towel-lined plate. Rehash the cycle with the leftover 2 eggs.

10. 4 . To serve, split the fresh tomato cuts between two plates. Top every fresh tomato with a couple of spinach leaves, 2 poached egg, and 2 loading tablespoons of the warm hollandaise.

11. Season with dark pepper and serve immediately.

Pegan-Friendly Granola

Ingredients:

1 cup raisins

1 cup sunflower seeds, unsalted

1 cup hazelnuts, chopped

1 cup pecans, chopped

4 tbsp coconut oil, melted

2 cup toasted coconut chips or pieces, unsweetened

2 tsp cinnamon, ground

1/2 cup cacao nibs

1-5 tbsp maple syrup, contingent upon your sweet tooth

Directions:

1. Preheat the stove to 450°F.

2. Just get an enormous rimmed baking sheet and line it with some material paper.

3. Add the nuts and seeds to the baking sheet and sprinkle them with coconut oil, cinnamon, and maple syrup.

4. Mix very well and guarantee everything is coated.
   Bake easily blend for 5 to 10 minutes and watch near not let the easily blend burn.

5. easy move from the broiler and easily blend in the cacao nibs, coconut chips,

and   raisins.
Can be delighted in quickly with a few
new leafy foods without dairy milk or
eaten once cooled.

6. When putting a easy way the granola,
   guarantee that it is totally cooled prior to
   setting it in an impenetrable holder.
7. It can just keep going for actually
   dependent upon one month.

Green Pineapple Smoothie

Ingredients

2 medium banana, peeled

 2 cup water

 2 cup canned full-fat coconut milk, divided

1 cup chopped dandelion greens

1 cup arugula

 2 cups chopped pineapple

Directions

1. Place dandelion greens, arugula, pineapple, banana, water and 1 cup coconut milk in a blender and easily blend until thoroughly combined.

2. Add remaining coconut milk while blending until desired texture is achieved.

Keto Vegetsuch Able Curry With Cauliflower Rice

Ingredients

.

- 2 shallot clove of

- .garlic

- .20 to 25 g ginger (2 piece)

- .450 g eggplant (2 eggplant) 200

- .g baby spinach

- .2 6 0 g tofu

- .

- .2 tbsp. lime juice

- .salt

- .pepper

- .4 0 g peanut kernel

- .20 to 25 g coriander green (0.6 bunch)

- .chilli pepper

- 250 g cauliflower

- 2 tbsp. peanut oil

- 2 tbsp. coconut oil

- .2 tsp. turmeric powder 2 tsp.

- .garam masala

- .2 tsp. curry powder 2 6 0 ml

- .vegetsuch able broth 450 ml coconut milk

Direction:

1. Peel and finely chop the shallot, garlic, coriander and ginger.

2. Easy cut the eggplant just into cubes after washing it.

3. Wash, dry and chop the spinach.

4. Easy cut the tofu just into cubes after draining it.

5. In a saucepan, melt the coconut oil and sauté parsley, garlic, and ginger.

6. Toss in the eggplant cubes and tofu, then season with turmeric, garam masala, and curry powder.
7. Allow the spinach to collapse before adding   it.

8. Pour the vegetsuch able stock over the top and bring to a boil for a few minutes.

9. Add the coconut milk, 2 tablespoon lime juice, salt, and pepper and easy cook for about 20 to 25 minutes over medium heat.

10. Meanwhile, coarsely chop the peanuts and chili peppers. **2 0.** At the end of cooking time, serve in 4 bowls drizzled with chili and peanuts.

Salmon-Stuffed Avocados Canned Salmon

is a precious pantry staple and a realistic manner to consist of heart-wholesome omega-three-wealthy fish to your diet. Here, we integrate it with avocados in an smooth no-prepare dinner dinner meal.

Ingredients

- 2 teaspoons mayonnaise
- 2 teaspoon Dijon mustard
- ⅛ teaspoon salt
- ⅛ teaspoon floor pepper
- 1 cup nonfat simple Greek yogurt
- 1 cup diced celery
- 2 tablespoons chopped sparkling parsley

72

- 2 tablespoon lime juice
- 2 (five ounce) cans salmon, tired, flaked, pores and skin and bones removed 2 avocados Chopped chives for garnish

Direction:

1. Combine yogurt, celery, parsley, lime juice, mayonnaise, mustard, salt, and pepper in a medium bowl; easily blend well.
2. Add salmon and easily blend well. Step 2 Halve avocados lengthwise and do a easy way with pits.
3. Scoop approximately 2 tablespoon flesh from every avocado 1 of right just into a small bowl.
4. Mash the scooped-out avocado flesh with a fork and stir just into the salmon aggregate.

5. Step three Fill every avocado 1 of with approximately 1 four cup of the salmon aggregate, mounding it on pinnacle of the avocado halves. Garnish with chives, if desired.

Sheet Pan Breakfast Fajitas

Ingredients:

- 4 teaspoons ground cumin

- 2 teaspoon ground paprika

- 1/2 teaspoon onion powder

- Kosher salt and freshly ground black pepper, to taste

- 6 large fresh eggs

- 2 avocado, halved, peeled, seeded and sliced

- 1/2 cup chopped fresh cilantro leaves

- 2 red bell pepper, thinly sliced

- 2 orange bell pepper, thinly sliced

- 2 green bell pepper, thinly sliced

- 2 tablespoons olive oil

- 2 tablespoon chili powder

- 2 tablespoon freshly squeezed lime juice

- 4 cloves garlic, minced

Directions:

1. Preheat oven to 450 degrees F. Lightly oil a baking sheet or coat with nonstick spray.
2. Place bell peppers in a single layer onto the prepared baking sheet.
3. Stir in olive oil, chili powder, lime juice, garlic, cumin, paprika and onion powder, and gently toss to combine; season with salt and pepper, to taste.
4. Place into oven and bake until tender, about 25 to 30 minutes.
5. Remove from oven and create 6 wells.
6. Add eggs, gently cracking the eggs throughout and keeping the yolk intact; season with salt and pepper, to taste.
7. Place into oven and bake until the egg whites have set, an additional 10 to 15 minutes.

8. Serve immediately, garnished with avocado and cilantro, if desired.

pegan Warm Breakfast Salad

Ingredients

- 1/2 tsp or more sea salt and black pepper each (to taste)

- 1/2 cup blueberries

- 4 fresh eggs

- red pepper flakes and cilantro to garnish

- 2 avocado (sliced)

- 7 cup chopped peeled butternut squash

- 1/2 c shopped red onion or shallot

- 4 tbsp olive oil or butter (divided)

- 2 2 ounces broccoli cole slaw salad mix

- 2 tbsp balsamic vinegar

- 2 tbsp water

- 1/2 tsp minced garlic or one garlic clove minced

Direction:

1. First peel and chop your veggies. Slice your avocado if you don't really want to wait till the end.
2. Place chopped squash in steamer on in microwave safe dish with 2 tbsp water.
3. Steam for 1 to 5 minutes or more. Depends on microwave power.
4. Cook until tender but not mushy.
5. Alternatively, roast squash on baking sheet at 450F for 20 to 25 minutes.
6. Remove, drain water, set aside.

7. In a small skillet, place 2 tbsp butter or oil.

8. Heat on medium high and add your onions.

9. Fry for 1 to 5 minutes or until onions easy start to brown a bit.

10. Next add in your slaw, garlic, salt/pepper, 2 tbsp water, and balsamic vinegar.

11. Mix all together in skillet.

12. Cover and let easy cook on medium for about 1-5 minutes.

13. Slaw will be slightly tender but not fully cooked.

14. Easily remove and place in bowl.

15. Add your squash and ½ cup berries to the bowl and toss.

16. Next fry your eggs in the same skillet.

17. Add another 1 tbsp of butter or oil on medium high heat.

18. Fry until crispy on outside and yolk is orange and set. 1 to 5 minutes or less depending on how you like your yolk.
19. Scoop slaw onto 1 to 5 plates or bowls.
20. Place fried egg on top of each.
21. Garnish with red pepper, 2 tbsp pumpkin seeds, cilantro, and any some extra salt/pepper.
22. Add sliced avocado on the side.

Pegan Diet Buddha Bowl

Ingredients

- Salt to Taste
- 20 to 25 cherry tomatoes
- 2 cup carrot sticks
- pumpkin seeds
- 450 grams button mushrooms sauteed
- 250 grams asparagus   sautéed
- 1 zucchini sliced
- 2 head iceberg lettuce
- ½ cup coloured cabbage optional
- 2 onions chopped fine
- 8 cloves garlic minced
- 1 teaspoon Red Chilli powder
- 6 boiled fresh eggs
- 1-5 cups quinoa boiled and sautéed
- 2 red capsicum |bell peppers

Direction:

1. Let us easy start chopping the veggies. Chop 2 onions fine, set aside Mince garlic fine , set aside Drain and Easy cut the mushrooms just into 1 or 1 ½ basically they have to be even sized. Chop the broccoli Peel the asparagus

2. By now the water for the eggs must be boiling.

3. Easily put the egg in a ladle and lower it in the boiling water.

4. I needed to boil 6 beggs.

5.

6. Let them boil for 20 to 25 minutes for a hardboiled eggs. When cooled peel and set aside.

7. Add the Ⓠuinoa and some salt to taste to the boiling water and mix well.

8. Just keep the flame on low and let the Ⓠuinoa cook.

9. The grains are cooked when you can see the Germ Check more about boiling quinoa in the link in the notes.

10. Add salt, garlic, some say about 4 tablespoon onions to the mushrooms, chilli powder and set aside.

11. Meanwhile, drain the eggs and in the same pan add the broccoli and a little water, salt and steam the broccoli.

12. In a sauce pan add the garlic, 2 teaspoon olive oil and roast till the raw smell goes away.

13. Add the asparagus and sauté till done. Set aside.

14. In the same pan add the mushroom and sauté till mushrooms are done. Set aside

15. Add 2 tablespoon oil add the rest of the garlic and onions and sauté.

16. Add the cooled quinoa and sauté. Set aside.

To assemble:

1. In a wide bowl add the lettuce leaves. Add 1-5 tblsp of sautéed quinoa, 2 tblsp mushrooms, the veggies, eggs and garnish with pumpkin seeds.

2. Serve immediately.

3. After all this, the bowl was over in a scant 20 to 25 minutes!

Smoked Salmon

Ingredients

- 1/2 cup Diamond Crystal kosher salt, about 2 ounces of any kosher salt

- 2 cup brown sugar

- ## 6 pounds salmon, trout or char

- Birch or maple syrup for basting

- BRINE

- 2 -quart cool water

Direction:

1. Mix the brine ingredients together, then place the fish in a non-reactive container

2. cover, and refrigerate.

3. This curing procedure removes part of the moisture from the interior of the fish while infusing it with salt, which aids in the preservation of the salmon.

4. Even for thin fillets of trout or pink salmon, you will really need to cure it for at least 4-4 ½ hours.

5. Large trout or char, as very well as pink, sockeye, and silver salmon, such require 8 hours in my experience.

6. A very thick chunk of king salmon might such require up to 40 to 45 hours to brine. If you leave it for longer than 48 hours, your fish will just get overly salty. If

the brine is not enough to coat the fish, double it.

7. Removing your fish from the brine and rinse it under cold running water before patting it dry.

8. Place the fillets skin-side down on a cooling rack.

9. This is best done beneath a high-speed ceiling fan or outside in a cool, breezy location. By "cool," I mean temperatures of 60°F or below.

10. Allow 2 to 4 hours for the fish to dry.

11. You really want the fish's surface to produce a pellicle, which is a glossy skin.

12. Many novice smokers overlook this step, but drying your cured, brined fish in a cool, windy location is critical to properly smoking it.

13. This lacquer-like covering, called a pellicle, is on the top of the fish and seals

it. It easily make it easy for the smoke to stick to. Just take it easy. Your fish won't just get bad because the brine is salty.

14. The fish can be chilled for a few hours after you just get your pellicle and then smoked if you want.

15. To making sure your fish doesn't stick to the smoker rack, easily put some oil on the skin. Even if this is hot smoking, you still do not really want it to really beeasy come too hot. Begin with a tiny fire and gradually increase the size.

16. If you do not gradually increase the temperature, the white albumin will "bleed" onto the meat.

17. With my smoker, I can adjust the temperature, so I easy start the process at

250°F to 250°F for up to an hour, then end at 250°F for another hour or two.

Overnight Oats With Almond Milk

Ingredients for Overnight Oats:

2 tbsp chia seeds
2 cup almond milk, unsweetened

2 cup oats, gluten-free

Toppings Ingredients:

2 tbsp coconut pieces, unsweetened
2 tbsp peanut butter, sugar-free

2 tbsp chocolate chips, 8 6 % or more

Directions:

1. Add every one of the elements for the short-term oats in a container and mix prior to adding a cover and setting it in the fridge.

2. Easy come morning, assuming the substance are excessively thick, add somewhat more almond milk until the consistency is at where you really need it to be.

3. Add your beloved fixings then enjoy.

Grilled Veggies With Creamy Cilantro And Mint Dip

Ingredients

- 2 -2 Green Chillies

- 2 " Ginger Piece

- 6 -6 Garlic Cloves

- 2 tsp Dry /Fresh Mint leaves

- 1-5 tbsp Olive Oil

- 1/2 tsp Turmeric Powder

- 7 tsp Salt or as per taste

- For Avocado Cilantro Dip

- 2 Avacado

- 2 Cup Fresh Cilantro

- 2 -2 Garlic Cloves

- 2 tbsp Lemon Juice

- 1-5 Green Chillies or as required

- 1-5 Mushrooms I used button mushrooms

- 2 Cup Cubed Red Onion

- 2 Cup Cubed Bell Peppers

- 8 -8 Cherry Tomatoes

- 1 Cup Thickly sliced Zucchini

- 1 tsp Raw Agave or any other plant based sweetner

- 2 tsp Red Chilli Powder optional or as required

- 1 tsp Cumin Powder

- 1 tsp Dry Mango Powder Pls see Notes

- Salt as per taste

Direction:

1. Wash and pat dry mushrooms. If using big mushrooms halve each , not really need to easy cut the small ones.

2. Take green chillies, garlic and ginger and grind to a fine paste.

3. Use mortar pestle.

4. If using fresh mint leaves grind with garlic and ginger.

5. In a bowl take oil, all the dry spice powders, prepared paste, sweetner, lemon juice and goat cheese.Mix well.

6. Add cubes veggies to the marinade and mix well.

7. Coat the veggie cubes with the marinade nicely.

8. Use hands for that.

9. Cover the bowl with cling film or lid and just keep in refrigerator for an hour.

10. Grill the veggies when ready to grill, arrange them on the skewers and grill for 20 to 25 minutes on a hot grill.

11. If using oven for grilling, preheat the oven to 200F and the grill on high for 20 to 25 minutes.

12. *Serve hot with the dip or green chutney.*

Orange French Toast

Ingredients:

- .1/2 Teaspoon grated nutmeg

- .4 Slices French bread

- .2 Tablespoon coconut oil

- 4 Very ripe bananas

- .2 Cup unsweetened nondairy milk

- .Zest and juice of 2 orange

- .2 Teaspoon ground cinnamon

Directions:

1. Easily blend the bananas, almond milk, orange juice and zest, cinnamon, and nutmeg and easily blend until smooth.
2. Dip the bread in the mixture for 5 to 10 minutes on each side.
3. While the bread soaks, simply eat a griddle or sauté pan over medium high heat.
4. Melt the coconut oil in the pan and swirl to coat.
5. Easy cook the bread slices until golden brown on both sides, about 5 to 10 minutes each.
6. Serve immediately.

Pegan Diet Detox Salad

Ingredients

- 1 cup pumpkin seeds
- 1 cup pomegranate seeds
- 2 cup green apple one medium thinly sliced
- orange peel, seeded and diced into small pieces
- 6 tablespoons extra virgin olive oil
- 4 tablespoons lime juice only use freshly squeezed, not the kind in a bottle
- 2 tablespoon almond butter
- 4 tablespoons honey optional

- 1 teaspoon salt

- 4 cups red cabbage very thinly sliced and loosely packed in the cup

- 4 cups kale thinly sliced kale, no stems and loosely packed in the cup
- 1/2 cup cilantro chopped just into small pieces, loosely packed. *hint I like to bunch my cilantro all together and cut with scissors.
- 2 cup yellow pepper diced just into small pieces *Note: you could also add red, orange, and green peppers too if you prefer.

Direction:

1. In a small jar that has a lid, mix together the olive oil, lime juice, almond butter, grated ginger, honey, and salt.

2. Shake until smooth and blended well.

3. Toss cabbage, kale, cilantro, apples, pumpkin seeds, yellow pepper, oranges,

103

and pomegranate seeds in a medium-sized bowl.

4. Drizzle the salad dressing over the veggies, stirring until the salad dressing is evenly distributed throughout the salad.

Berry Power Smoothie

Ingredients: .

- .1 cup baby spinach

- .2 tablespoons unsalted almond butter

- 5 cups coconut milk or unsweetened nut milk

- 1/2 cup frozen blueberries

- .1/2 cup frozen strawberries

Directions:

1. Place every one of the fixings just into a blender and heartbeat until all around consolidated, around 2 minute.

2. Pour just into a glass and appreciate immediately.

Grain-Free Nutty Granola

Ingredients:

- 2 tablespoon maple syrup

- .2 teaspoon alcohol-free vanilla extract

- 2 .teaspoon ground cinnamon, or to taste

- .1/2 teaspoon sea salt or Himalayan salt

- 4 cups chopped raw walnuts or pecans

- .2 cup raw almonds, sliced

- .1 cup seeds, toasted or roasted unsalted sunflower, sesame, or shelled pumpkin

107

- .1/2 cup unsweetened coconut flakes

- .1 cup coconut oil or unsalted grass-fed butter, melted

.

Directions:

1. Preheat stove to 450°F. 2. Line a rimmed baking sheet with material paper or foil.

2. Add the pecans, almonds, seeds, and coconut chips to an enormous bowl.
3. In a such different bowl, easily blend the oil in with the maple syrup, vanilla, cinnamon, and salt.
4. Pour over the nut blend, throwing to coat. 4. Spread the combination equally on the

pre-arranged baking sheet and prepare
until brilliant brown, around 25 to 30

Steamed Fish Fillet

Ingredients

.

- 2 shallot

- .1 tuber fennel

- .120 g small carrots

- .2 tbsp. classic vegetable broth salt

- pepper

- .1 small lime

- .150g pangasius fillet

- 4 stems flat leaf parsley

Direction:

1. Finely chop the shallot.

2. Wash the carrot and fennel and easy cut them just into thin sticks.

3. In a covered pan, hsimply eat the broth. Add the shallot, fennel and carrot and easy cook for about 4 minutes. Season with salt to taste.

4. Wash and dry the fish fillet, place it on the vegetables and gently salt.

5. Cover and easy cook for 20 to 25 minutes over low heat.

6. Meanwhile wash the parsley, shake it, easy move the leaves with a large knife

and   chop   finely.

7. Once the fish is cooked, squeeze it on top half a lime if you like.

8. Season with salt and pepper to taste, then garnish with parsley and serve.

Quinoa Pegan Salad Bowl

Ingredients

For the salad

- 1 cup Cabbage purple/red, shredded

- 1 cup black bean cooked and drained

- 2 cup quinoa cooked

- 2 cup Spinach baby leaves, packed

- 1 medium cucumber

- 1/2 cup Onion chopped

For The Dressing:

- 4 tsp Lemon juice

- black pepper powder to taste

- 2 tsp miso paste (gluten free)

Direction:

1. wash and cook quinoa to get 2 cup of cooked quinoa

2. Fluff and set it aside to cool.

3. Collect the ingredients for the salad, wash and drain all.

4. Chop the onions, cucumbers and shred the cabbage.

5. Add these to the salad bowl arranging them on the such different sides of the bowl.

6. Drain and add the black beans to the bowl.

7. Add the now cooled quinoa.

8. Whisk the miso, the lemon juice, the salt and pepper together to form the dressing.

9. Pour the dressing over the salad, toss if desired and enjoy.

Perfectly Roasted Parsnip Chips

Ingredients

1/7 teaspoon nutmeg

2 teaspoon cinnamon

6 large parsnips, peeled and easy cut
diagonally just into thin slices

4 tablespoons olive oil

Directions

1. Preheat oven to 450°F. Spray a large
    baking sheet with cooking spray.

2. In a large bowl, combine parsnips, olive
    oil, and spices and stir to coat.

3. Arrange parsnips on baking sheet in a single layer and easy cook for 25 to 30 minutes.

4. easy move from oven and turn on broiler.

5. Broil chips for 5 to10 minutes.

6. Serve warm or at room temperature.

Super Tasty Ginger Garlic Walnuts

Ingredients

1/2 teaspoon onion powder

1/2 teaspoon garlic powder

4 cups shelled walnuts

2 tablespoons coconut oil

1/2 cup maple syrup

2 teaspoon ground ginger

2 teaspoon curry powder

1 teaspoon cayenne

Directions

1. Place coconut oil in a 1-5 quart slow cooker, turn on high, and allow oil to melt.
2. While oil is melting, mix maple syrup, ginger, curry powder, cayenne, onion powder, and
3. garlic powder together in a small bowl.

4. Once oil has melted, add walnuts to slow cooker and stir.

5. Add maple syrup mixture to slow cooker, and stir until nuts are evenly coated.

6. Cover and easy cook on high for 25 to 30 minutes.

7. Easily remove cover and easy cook for an additional 25 to 30 minutes, until nuts are

dry.

8. Cool and store in airtight containers in a cool, dry place for up to several weeks.

Caprese Salad With Grilled Flank Steak

Ingredients

- 2 tablespoon olive oil
- salt and ground black pepper to taste
- 2 (6.6 ounce) bag butter lettuce mix
- 2 tablespoons balsamic vinegar, or to taste
- olive oil, or to taste
- 2 tomatoes, diced
- 2 (4 ounce) ball fresh mozzarella, cut just into 2 -inch cubes
- 1/2 cup coarsely chopped fresh basil
- 2 clove garlic, minced, or more to taste

122

- 2 tablespoon olive oil
- 2 pound flank steak
- 2 clove garlic, minced

Directions

1. Mix tomatoes, mozzarella, basil, 2 clove minced garlic, and 2 tablespoon olive oil in a bowl; toss to coat. Cover bowl and refrigerate.
2. Preheat an outdoor grill for medium-high hsimply eat and lightly oil the grate.
3. Place steak in a large resealable bag; add 2 clove minced garlic, 2 tablespoon olive oil, salt, and pepper.
4. Seal the bag and distribute the oil mixture over the steak.

5. Cook the steak on the preheated grill to your desired degree of doneness, about 5 to 10 minutes per side for medium.

6. An instant-read thermometer inserted into the center should read 250 degrees F (60 degrees C). Let stand for 5 to 10 minutes before thinly slicing across the grain.

7. Divide lettuce onto 4 serving plates; drizzle about 4 teaspoons balsamic vinegar and 4 teaspoons olive oil onto each lettuce portion.

8. Top each salad with 1/2 the steak and 1/2 the fresh tomato mixture.

Rainbow Fruit Salad

Ingredients

- 1/2 cup orange juice

- 2 tablespoons lemon juice

- 4 tablespoons maple syrup

- 1/2 teaspoon ground ginger

- 1/7 teaspoon ground nutmeg

- 2 large mango, peeled and diced

- 2 cups fresh blueberries

- 2 cup sliced bananas

- 2 cups halved strawberries

- 2 cups halved seedless grapes

- 2 cup peeled, sliced nectarines

125

- 1 cup peeled, sliced kiwi fruit

Directions

1. In a large bowl, gently toss together mango, blueberries, bananas, strawberries, grapes, nectarines, and kiwi.

2. In a small bowl, stir together orange juice, lemon juice, maple syrup, ginger, and nutmeg; mix well.

3. Chill fruit until needed, for up to 4-4 ½ hours.

4. Just before serving, pour orange sauce over fruit and toss gently to coat.

Shaved Fennel Salad With Orange Sections And Toasted Hazelnuts

Ingredients

- ½ cup orange juice

- 2 tablespoons extra-virgin olive oil

- 2 tablespoon orange zest

- 6 large oranges, peeled

- 4 medium bulbs fennel, finely sliced

- 2 teaspoon finely chopped hazelnuts

127

Directions

1. With a small paring knife, easily remove each section of the oranges and slice aeasy way membrane.

2. Form a mound of sliced fennel on each serving plate and arrange oranges on top.

3. Sprinkle with nuts, then drizzle with orange juice and olive oil.

4. Finish with a sprinkle of zest.

Arugula And Fennel Salad With Pomegranate And Chicken

Ingredients

- 2 large navel oranges, peeled and sliced just into small pieces

- 2 large pomegranate, seeds and surrounding flesh only

- 4 cups arugula

- 1 cup thinly sliced fennel

- 6 tablespoons olive oil, divided

- 2 pound boneless, skinless chicken breast

- ½ teaspoon salt

- ½ teaspoon ground black pepper, divided

129

Directions

1. simply eat 2 tablespoon olive oil in large nonstick skillet over medium heat.

2. Season both sides of chicken with salt and $1/2$ teaspoon pepper.

3. Add chicken to the skillet.

4. Cover and easy cook until just cooked through, 5 to 10 minutes on each side.

5. Transfer chicken to a cutting board and let cool.

6. Easy cut the chicken just into bite-sized pieces.

7. Add orange pieces and pomegranate seeds to a large bowl.

8. Add arugula, fennel slices, remaining olive oil, and remaining pepper.

9. Toss to coat and serve immediately.

Pork Cacciatore

Ingredients:

2 small onion, diced

2 garlic clove, minced

2 tablespoon olive oil

1/2 teaspoon pepper

1 teaspoon salt

4 lbs. pork chops

2 teaspoon dried oregano

2 cup beef broth

4 tablespoon fresh tomato paste

15 oz can tomato, diced

2 cups mushrooms, sliced

Directions:

1. Warmth oil in a pan over medium-high heat.

2. Add pork chops in pan and easy cook until brown on both the sides.
3. Transfer pork chops just into a pot.

4. Pour remaining ingredients over the pork chops.

5. Cover then easy cook on low flame for 2 hours.

6. Serve and enjoy.

Conclusion

The pegan diet is based on paleo and vegan principles — though it encourages some meat consumption. It emphasizes whole foods, especially vegetables, while largely prohibiting gluten, dairy, most grains, and legumes.

It's rich in many nutrients that can promote optimal health but may be too restrictive for many people. You can give this diet a easy try to see how your body responds. If you're already paleo or vegan and are interested in modifying your diet, the pegan diet may be easier to adjust to.

To sum up, the Pegan diet is not the easiest and least-demanding one. It emphasizes the importance of plant food, which is basically rather nutritious and is linked to inflammation reduction. Additionally, healthy fats from plants and fish can improve your heart health. Also, it is not recommended to avoid gluten and dairy unless you have specific allergies and intolerances. Foreover, sticking to this eating may be a rather bothersome process, so you might be forced to spend ⬚uite a lot of time in the supermarket choosing the foods that would fit this diet. Many of the products you would need, such as grass-fed meat, are pretty expensive. So, the Pegan diet might actually work for you, but it's also demanding and, in addition, not all of its guidelines are scientifically grounded and must be strictly followed if you really want to lose weight and enhance your health.

The pegan diet gets a few things right with its emphasis on eating more fruits, vegetables, healthy fats and actually lean proteins. But the idea that everyone can or should avoid dairy, grains and legumes is not realistic nor is it supported by scientific evidence. There is also no evidence to support the idea that people without a gluten allergy or intolerance should avoid gluten. Pegan's emphasis on minimally processed and organic foods is not practical for many people who can't afford all-organic diets, and also requires that followers have a more-than-typical amount of time availsuch able for cooking and planning meals—a luxury many people don't have. The concept of this diet, combined with its number of restrictive rules, will likely make it hard to follow long-term and add to confusion about what to eat and why.

www.ingramcontent.com/pod-product-compliance
Lightning Source LLC
Chambersburg PA
CBHW050731030426
42336CB00012B/1516